The GET-WELL BOOK

Fun and Games To Help You Feel Better

Edited by Tina Hacker
Illustrated by John Overmyer

Hallmark Editions

"Do you remember..." and "A shipping tycoon..." from *The Sound of Laughter* by Bennett Cerf. Copyright © 1970 by Doubleday & Company, Inc. "You certainly seemed..." and "The whole neighborhood..." from *Laugh Day* by Bennett Cerf. Copyright © 1965 by Bennett Cerf. Published by Doubleday & Company, Inc. All reprinted by permission of Doubleday & Company, Inc. "The Germ" from *Verses From 1929 On* by Ogden Nash. Copyright 1935 by The Curtis Publishing Company. Reprinted by permission of Little, Brown and Company and J M Dent & Sons Limited. "Wonder Drugs" and "Medicine in Prehistoric Times" from *It All Started With Hippocrates* by Richard Armour. Copyright © 1966 by Richard Armour. Used with permission of McGraw-Hill Book Company. "Chicken Soup or 'Jewish Penicillin'" from *Everything But Money* by Sam Levenson. Copyright 1946, 1966 by Sam Levenson. Used with permission of Simon & Schuster, Inc.

© 1976, Hallmark Cards, Inc., Kansas City, Missouri. Printed in the United States of America. Library of Congress Catalog Card Number: 75-6208. Standard Book Number: 87529-453-7.

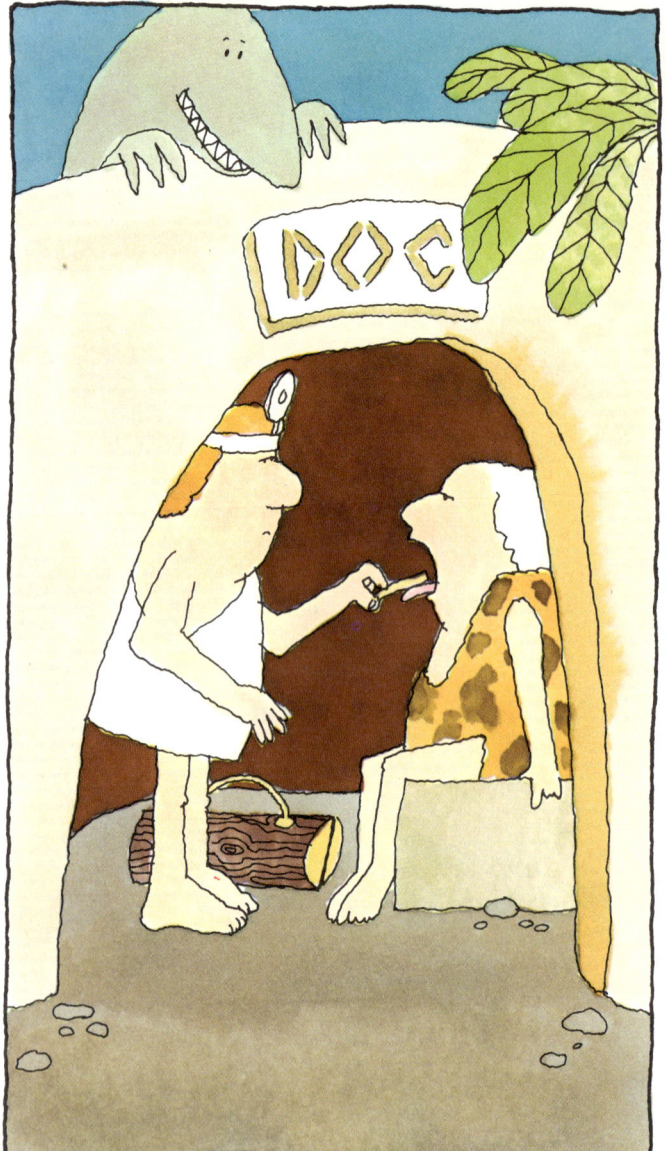

Medicine in Prehistoric Times

Medicine began with the dawn of history. In fact it began shortly before dawn, at about 3:00 A.M., when the first Stone Age doctor was routed from his bed to attend a patient who thought he was dying. Transportation being none too good (this being before the invention of the wheel), by the time the doctor arrived the patient was well.

During the Stone Age the most common complaints were gallstones, kidney stones, and stumbling over stones. Some complaints could be heard for blocks. There being no telephones, the doctor had to be summoned by going to his cave and knocking. Since knocking on the mouth of the cave made no sound and knocking on the stones around the mouth of the cave was hard on the knuckles, it was often necessary to resort to some other way of getting the doctor's attention. The usual way was to throw a stone into the opening. If it lit near the doctor, he would hear it and know someone needed help. If it hit the doctor, he would need help himself.

The doctor's little black bag was at first a little brown bag, since it was made of tree bark. A doctor with a friendly bedside manner often made a joke of this as he entered the sickroom. "My bark is worse than my bite," he would say, thereupon laughing so uproariously that it was hard to believe he had used the same witticism as an icebreaker on six previous

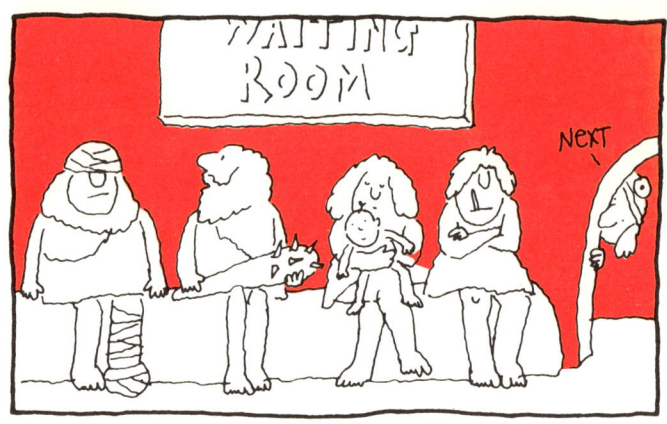

calls that day....

Some doctors had their office in their home — in other words, in the same cave or in a small cave attached to the main cave but with its own outside entrance. They could write off this part of their home as a business expense, even though it could also be used as a guest bedroom.

Most doctors, however, had their office in a cave downtown or in a medico-dental cliff, honeycombed with caves. Since there were no old magazines, the doctor's waiting room was an even drearier place than it is now. Patients had nothing with which to divert themselves, and often sat there for hours, whittling a soft stone with a hard stone. For the most part, though, they passed the time much as they do today, looking furtively at the other patients and wondering what was the matter with them....

Richard Armour

Your Personal Autograph Cast

Announcing the world's first portable, personal autograph cast! A cast that does not cost you an arm and a leg. Here is the perfect place for all those witty comments and cute pictures you've been saving up for just a chance like this!

Directions: 1. Please sign or draw below.
2. After ten weeks, a physician may remove this cast from the book.

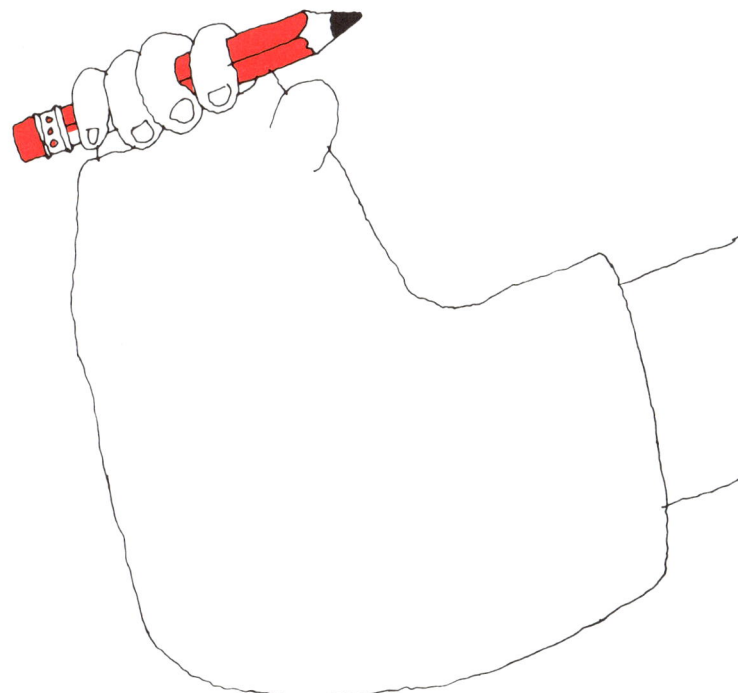

Have I Got an Answer for You
(Don't You Wish You Never Asked?)

Tired of telling everybody how you feel, if you feel better, or if you feel at all? Here's the solution for you. When someone inquires about the state of your health, just hold up this book, point to the right answer and grunt.

YOU DON'T LOOK SO GOOD YOURSELF...

Where's the truck that ran over me?

I MAY BE CONTAGIOUS.

Do you want the short or long version?

I'm in stitches all the time.

i feel lousy, thank you.

YOU ATE EVERYTHING THERE IS-- YOU CAN GO NOW.

EVEN THE DOG CAN'T PRONOUNCE WHAT I'VE GOT.

THE CURE IS WHAT'S KILLING ME..

I'M ALLERGIC TO FREE MEDICAL ADVICE.

Scramblers
(Word Games Even Shakespeare Would Enjoy)

Directions:
1. See if you can make four ordinary words out of the scrambled words next to each question.
2. Solve the riddle by unscrambling the circled letters.

1. How did the barnyard
   chick receive the news
   that you got sick?
   Answer: With a _____

   gluha _ ◯ _ _ _
   estwe ◯◯ _ _ _
   tnaek _ _ ◯ _ _
   cikuq ◯◯ _ _ _

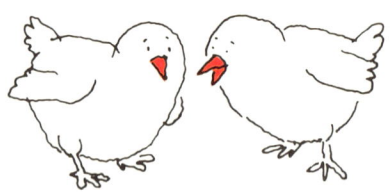

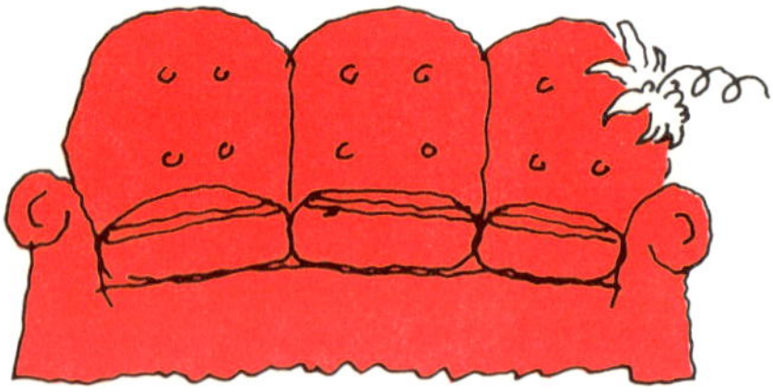

2. Here's some good advice
   for you: do what all
   upholsterers do.
   Answer: _____

   ecrkw _ ◯ _ ◯ _
   kirpe _ _ _ ◯◯
   icoev ◯ _ _ _ ◯
   kcokn _ _ ◯ _ _

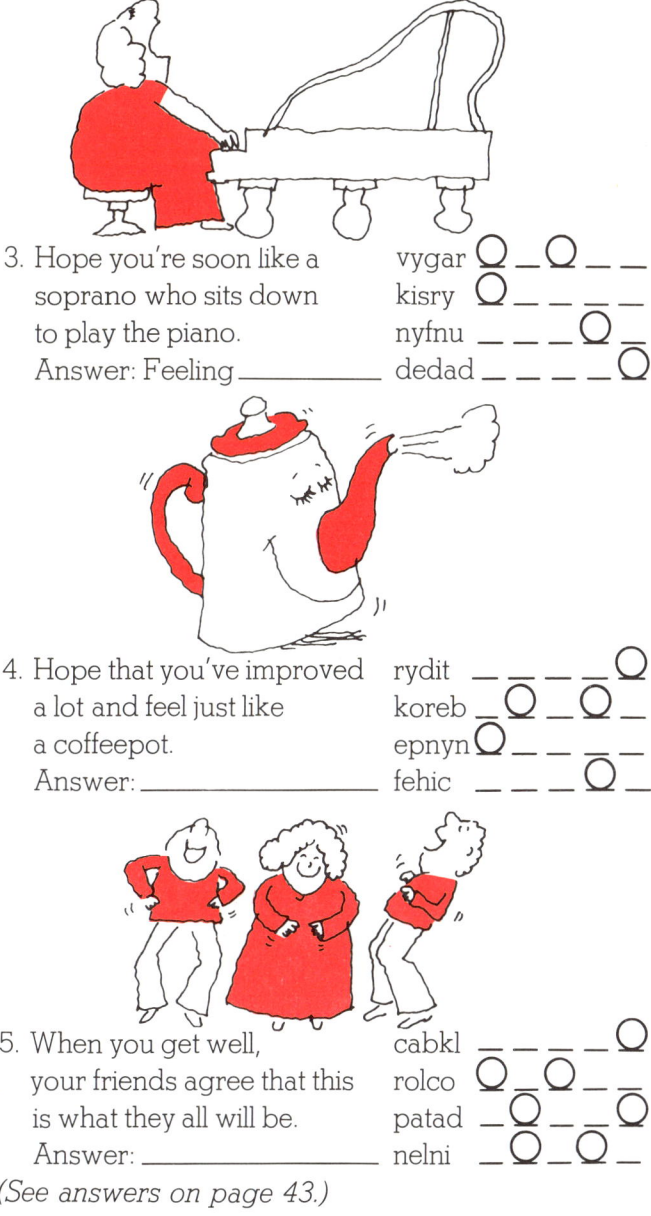

3. Hope you're soon like a soprano who sits down to play the piano.
Answer: Feeling _____

vygar ○_○___
kisry ○____
nyfnu ___○_
dedad ____○

4. Hope that you've improved a lot and feel just like a coffeepot.
Answer: _____

rydit ____○
koreb _○_○_
epnyn○___○_
fehic ___○_

5. When you get well, your friends agree that this is what they all will be.
Answer: _____

cabkl ____○
rolco ○_○__
patad _○__○
nelni _○_○_

(See answers on page 43.)

7

Help the Doctor Find the Patient

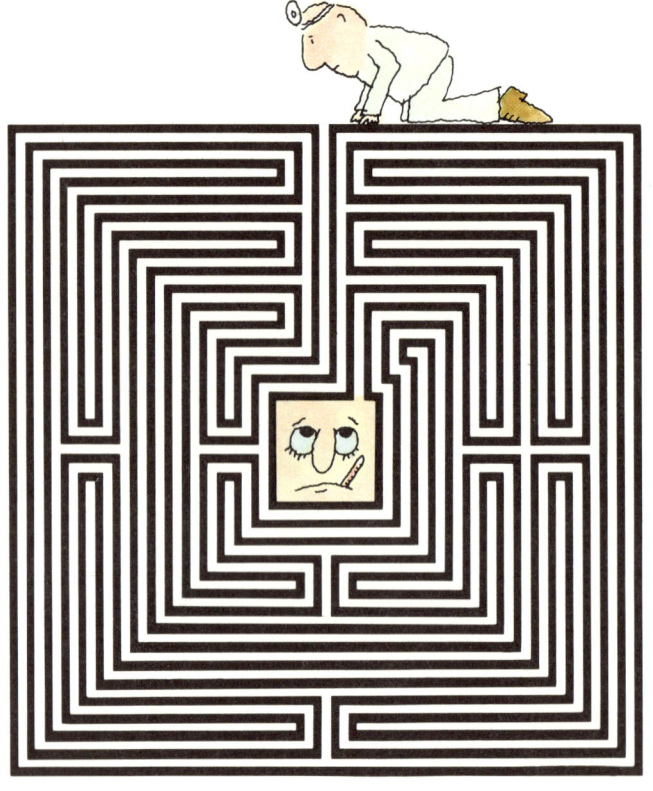

With pencil, find path between doctor and patient. Time yourself. Erase line. Have your doctor work maze. Time him (or her). If time is longer, find new doctor. (After all, doc had an erased line to follow.) If doctor completes maze in record time, send him (or her) an entertainment bill for $10.

Mystery Thrillers to Solve

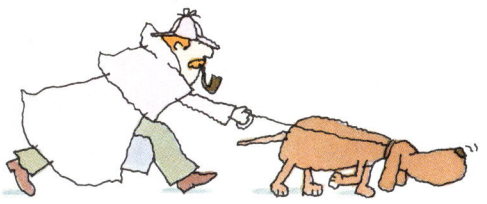

(1) *The Case of the Relentless Racers;
or, Truth Wins Out*

Two cars were racing a distance of fifty miles. Sam and Sadie were driving a new, low-slung racer, and Pat McGee was sporting a souped-up 1910 Stanley Steamer. There were no witnesses to the race and both claimed the victory. When Sharp, the private eye, was called in on the case, he said, "Sam and Sadie, you are lying!" How did he know?

(2) *The Case of the Panhandler Queen;
or, Think Twice Before You Judge!*

The Amalgamated American Panhandlers were having their annual convention at Freightville to make plans for their new membership drive. Someone suggested they sponsor a beauty contest. Sharp was called in to select the judges. After a moment, he shook his head sadly and said, "None of you have the qualifications to judge this contest!" What brought him to this conclusion?

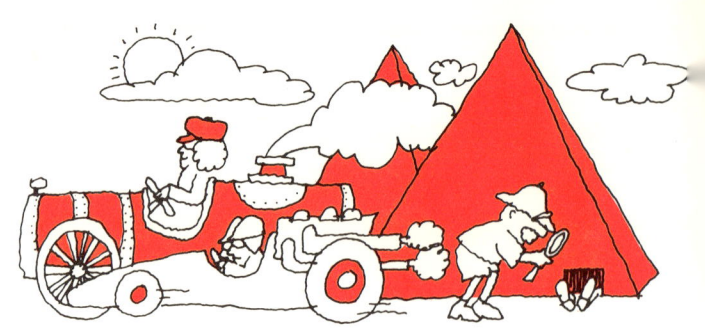

(3) *The Case of the Halting Horse;
or, It Just Takes Horse Sense!*

In the fifth race at Upsan Downs, Misery, a twenty-to-one favorite, was coming into the stretch a good six lengths ahead of the field. Suddenly he came to a halt and trotted across the finish line a weak sixth. The irate owner, sure that the race had been fixed, called on Sharp to investigate. Sharp surveyed the situation, then pointed to the owner and said, "You are at fault here. It was impossible for this horse to finish first and you should know why." Do you know why?

(4) *The Case of the Stolen Gems;
or, Justice Shines Through*

Private eye Sharp had been called in to question three suspects in the disappearance of the priceless South African collection of rare gems that had been on display at Spiffany's Jewelry Salon.

"I was at de ballet all afternoon," claimed Shifty Sullivan.

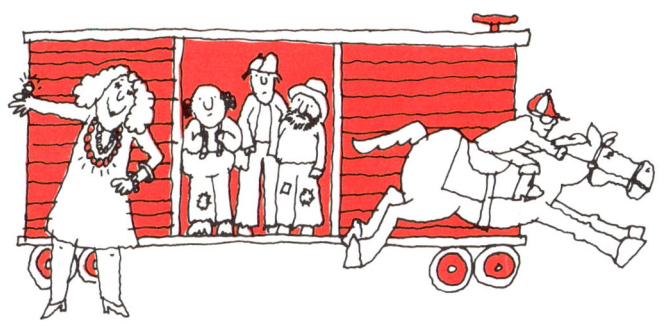

"Me? I was visitin' de Art Museum," maintained Muscles McTwitch. The last suspect, Sylvia Sweetsoul, said, "Why, little ole me? I spent the afternoon with my best friend." Instantly Sharp said, "Aha! You, Sylvia Sweetsoul, are the thief!" How did Sharp come so quickly to this conclusion?

(5) *The Quest of the Lost Pyramid;
or, Mummy's the Word*

Will and Phil went on a desert expedition to find King Be-Bop's lost pyramid. When after a month Will and Phil had not returned, Sharp was called in on the case. His investigation showed that two shady characters had just come back with the treasure. When he questioned them, the two claimed to have found Will and Phil's broken compass in the sand. "Will and Phil must have lost their way," they said. Sharp whipped out his gun. "That's impossible. I know they met with foul play." How did he know?

(See answers on page 43.)

G-B* GUIDE

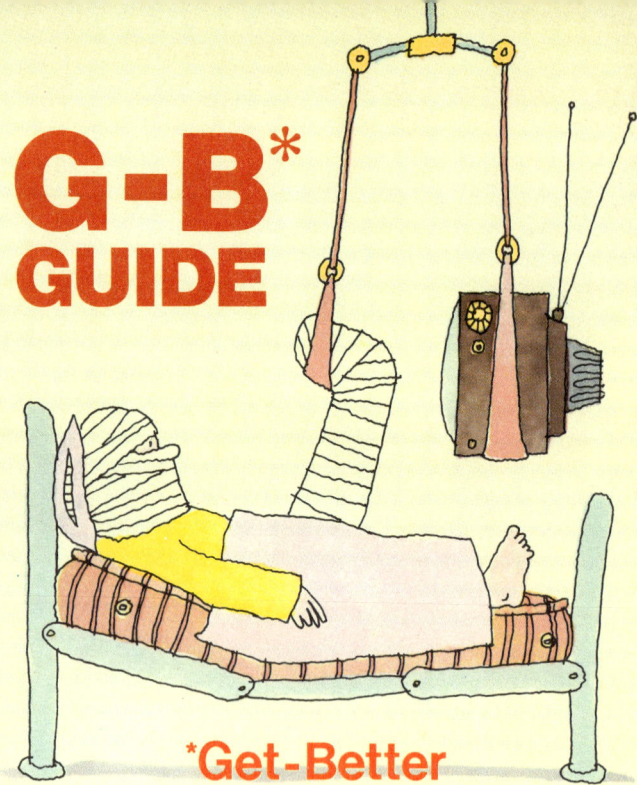

*Get-Better

Afternoon

5:00 ❻❽ **COLONEL ARMADILLO**
Kiddie Show
The colonel demonstrates the evils of alcohol by chugging a quart of gin, chasing an attractive girl around the set, kicking over all the props and smashing a $30,000 color camera with a sledgehammer. (Black & White)

5:30 ❻❽ **DR. JOE SISTERS**
Noted psychiatrist cures a watch repairman's tic.

6:00 ❺ **MICROSCOPE**
Lonely amoeba is fed up at home and splits.

Evening

6:30 ❷❻⓭ **INCARCERATED**
Drama
Refreshingly candid story of John Shaw, acquitted for a crime he really committed, and his struggle to convince friends, business associates and his own lawyer of his guilt.

12

Evening

❽ MEAT AND THE PRESS
Panel of distinguished newsmen interview Bess, a guernsey cow.

7:00 **❷ ❻ ⓳ MILD KINGDOM**
You'd love a little termite who wouldn't chew, wouldn't you? A look into the fascinating world of termites. Watch a small colony of these industrious creatures make mincemeat of an $85,000 home.

7:30 **❷ ❾ ⓳ THE DOORKNOBS**
Drama
A visit with America's favorite millionaire family on their 30,000-acre egg ranch. Laugh and cry with Jean-girl as she learns that life is just an elaborate chicken joke.

8:00 **❻ ⓳ MOVIE OF THE WEAK**
Tragicomedy
"My World Turns Counterclockwise." Low-budget ($37) film shot in 1931. Given new life on television. Hackneyed plot (boy meets girl, boy and girl fall in love, boy marries girl, girl is found to have rare, curable disease). Low-grade acting (cast all high-school dropouts). Poor location (filmed in the dark in subbasement of bus station). Despite its obvious flaws, "My World Turns Counterclockwise" has become a modern classic of the "Waddles the Duck Is Pigeon-toed" genre. EXCELLENT (6 hrs. 37 min.)

9:00 **❷ ❺ METER MAID**
Crime Drama
Dauntless policewoman Mary Glotz continues her relentless one-woman battle against the forces of overtime parkers. In this episode Mary tickets her husband's car. He ends up in traffic court. Mary smiles. She ends up in divorce court.

10:00 **❼ MS. OLD-AGE AMERICA BEAUTY PAGEANT**
First annual presentation direct from Social Security headquarters in Baltimore, Md. One elderly lady will be chosen to represent her country at senior citizen centers around the world. Contestants will be judged on the basis of personality, poise, the quality of their dentures, the number of grandchildren and the makeup of their stock portfolios. Winner receives a lifetime membership in the School of Ballroom Dancing and a two-week part-time job.

Feel Better — Get Well! Your Best Bet Now and Always!
— Adv.

11:00 **❷ ❺ ❼ ❻ ⓳ ❽**
FEEL BETTER — GET WELL
Presentation of latest medical findings which indicate the reason more people are not feeling well is because they are sick. Evidence indicates that people feel better as soon as they get well.

A Unique Personality Quiz
To Reveal the *Real* You

1. What kind of animal would you like to be? (check one)
   - ☐ Goat
   - ☐ Rhinoceros
   - ☐ Skunk
   - ☐ Fox
   - ☐ Lion
2. What is your favorite residence?
   - ☐ Southern Mansion
   - ☐ Coed Dormitory
   - ☐ Lighthouse
   - ☐ Neighborhood Bar
   - ☐ Doghouse
3. Which of these books would you rather have if you were marooned on a desert island?
   - ☐ The Care and Cleaning of Fig Leaves
   - ☐ How to Train a Sea Gull
   - ☐ The Life and Loves of Cleopatra
   - ☐ Plantation Farming
   - ☐ How to Build Your Own TV Set
4. What do you want more than anything in the world?
   - ☐ A pet yak
   - ☐ A vacation
   - ☐ A man
   - ☐ Money
   - ☐ A woman

(See answers on page 43.)

Nurse Josephine's Jolly Page

A man went to the hospital to visit a friend who was recuperating from a tonsillectomy. As he started up in the elevator the operator asked, "What floor?"

The visitor thought for a moment, then brightened and said crisply, "Men's tonsils, please."

C. Kennedy

"You certainly seemed fascinated by that medical magazine in my waiting room," observed a doctor as he prepared to examine a patient. "Indeed I was," agreed the patient. "The issue you have out there announces the discovery of ether."

"Medicine won't help you any," the doctor told the elderly patient. "What you need is a complete rest and a change of living. Get away to some quiet country place for a month. Go to bed early, eat more roast beef, drink plenty of good rich milk, and smoke just one cigar a day."

A month later the patient walked into the doctor's office. He looked like a new man and the doctor told him so.

"Yes, Doctor, your advice certainly did the business. I went to bed early and did all the other things you told me. But say, Doctor, that one cigar a day almost killed me. It's no joke starting to smoke at my age."

Activity Games

HIDDEN TREASURE

Directions: This will add fun and excitement to the lives of those people who are looking in on you as well as test your imaginative ability. The object of this game is to hide items around your bed — such as thermometers, spoons, doctor's bag, bedpans — and see how long it takes your opponent (or nurse or physician) to find them.

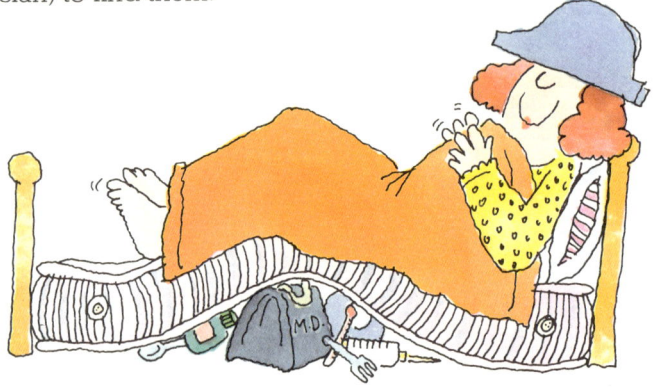

Scoring: 8 to 10 minutes — excellent.
         5 to 7 minutes — good.
         3 to 4 minutes — average.
         Below 3 minutes — poor. Hand in your Captain Hook Honorary Pirate's badge. You can't hide anything!

for One or More

TOE TOSS

Directions: Ask your doctor, nurse, wife, husband, friend, etc., to cut out three cardboard rings, making the circumference about the size of the rim of a cup. Propping yourself up in bed, see how many times you can throw the ring around your big toe or toes (easiest done with covers removed).

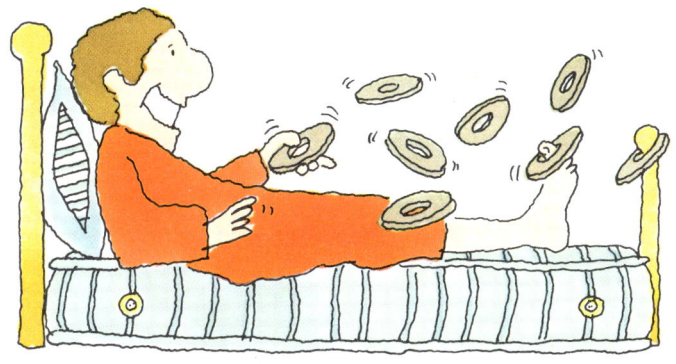

Scoring: 10 out of 10 — excellent or you are cheating. Lean back and try again.
7 to 9 — good.
4 to 6 — you need practice.
1 to 3 — you are not the athletic type.
Better luck at the next game.

Confidential

(The Contents of This Page Will Self-Destruct If They Are Dropped in the Sink)

At last! Here is your chance to escape from your hospital or sickroom. CAUTION! Do it right away with the help of these two pages. While you're formulating an escape route, here is a map of a typical hospital to test your ability to find the way out. If you are at home, at mother's, or in a bus station, disregard this map. In that case, ask the nearest five-year-old to direct you to an exit, look for an obvious clue like a front door, and/or buy a ticket on the next bus.

Here, also, are some cutout disguises to aid you in your plan of escape. One reminder before you leave, hospital nighties are a dead giveaway, if you know what we mean.

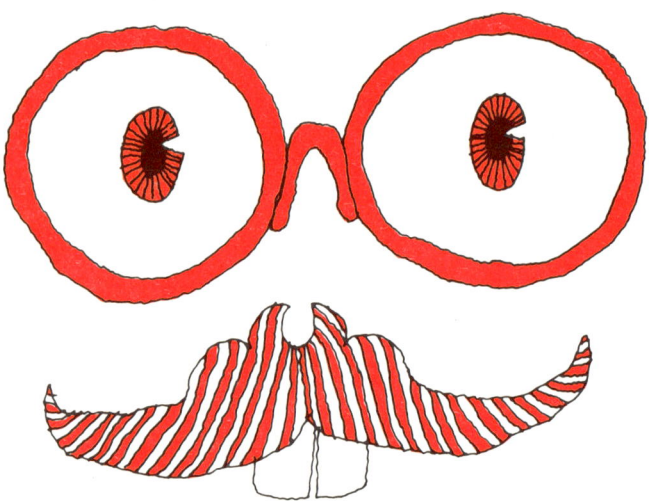

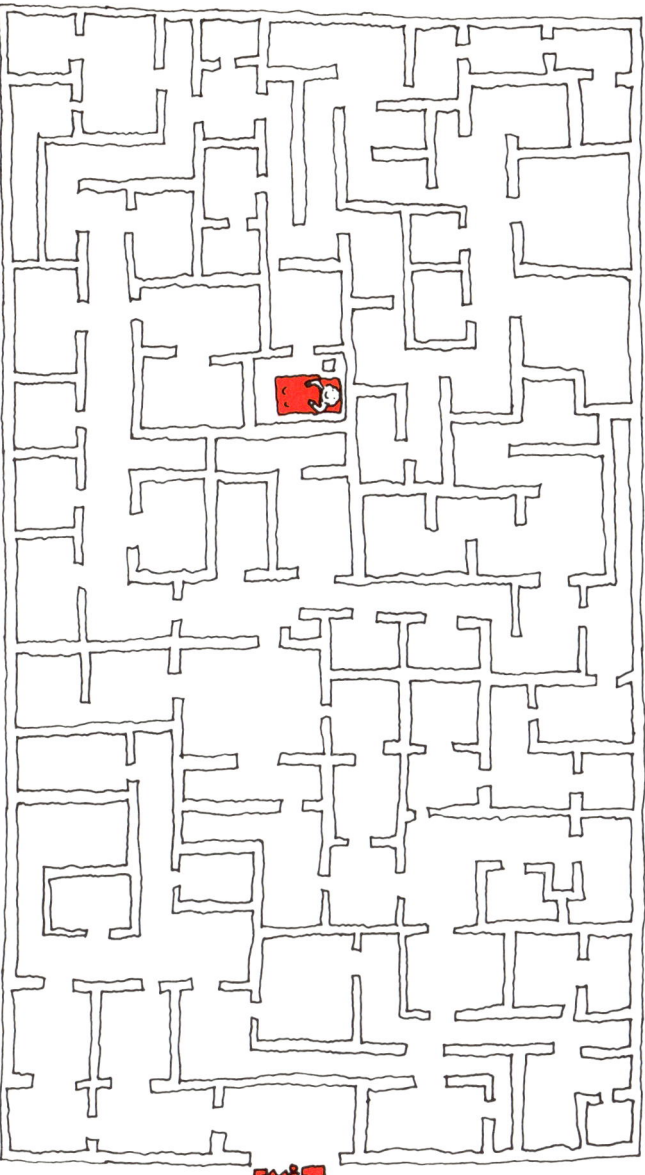

How to Spend Your Time While Recuperating

1. Wiggle your ears in 4/4 time.
2. Memorize all the verses of "Jingle Bells."
3. Try to recall the names of ten current spies on TV.
4. Count the number of zeros in one million billion trillion.
5. Listen to radio commercials and count the number of times "new" is used.
6. Try to imagine Napoleon Bonaparte as a little boy.
7. Learn the Morse code.
8. Take your pulse.
9. Enter a soap contest.
10. Hand-color your drinking straw.
11. Write a singing commercial for the U.S. Steel Corporation.
12. Try to name the seven dwarfs.
13. Answer an ad on how to make BIG money at home.
14. Practice saying: rubber baby-buggy bumpers.
15. Now try repeating it real fast.
16. Yell and count the seconds it takes for someone to come.
17. Take your watch apart.
18. Try to remember one of your high school cheers.
19. Write your congressman and ask him what he's doing.
20. Answer a want ad for a job for which you're completely unqualified.

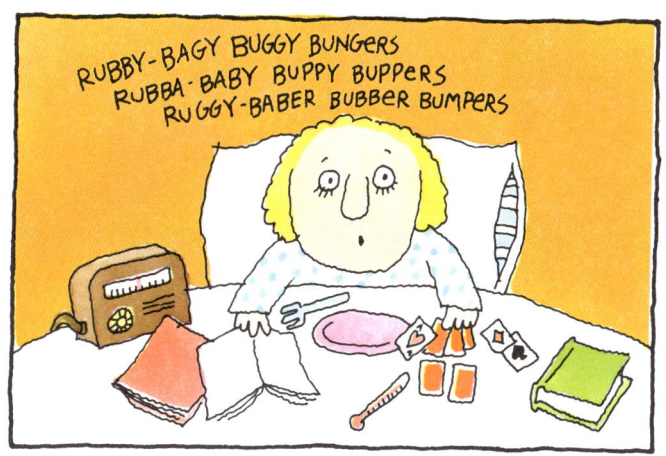

21. Try to imagine Lassie as a little pup.
22. Try to name the fifty states.
23. Try to find out from your nurse how you're getting along.
24. Practice cheating at cards.
25. Memorize the Top 40 songs backwards.
26. Memorize the Gettysburg Address.
27. Work out the square root of 11,233.
28. Learn to tie a bowline knot.
29. Write a hit song on your punch-dial telephone.
30. Name all the movies you can starring Humphrey Bogart.
31. See how long you can go without blinking.
32. Say the alphabet backwards.
33. Read a medical book and count the number of symptoms you have.
34. Give thanks for the symptoms you *don't* have.
35. Make up ten new names for the common cold.

The All-Purpose Pill Directory

After you've taken the little red pills, the long yellows, and the oblong pills with the pink stripes — you might try some of these!

Basepill — the all-American pill.
Combination Pill — for whatever you've got; or just name it, it's here.
Sugar Pill — tastes like a mint, works like a mint, costs a mint.
Salt Pill — when it pains, it pours.
Doctor Pill — to be taken before the bill comes.
Water Pill — for that clogged-up feeling.
Slow Pill — relief is just fifteen hours, thirty-six minutes and four seconds away. (Or twenty thousand miles, whichever comes first.)
Dime Pill — reminds you to feed the meter while you're waiting in the doctor's office.
Smile Pill — for a pained expression.
X-Rated Pill — to be taken by adults only.
Cracked Pill — for people who are mixed up about which pill to take.

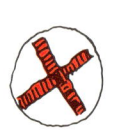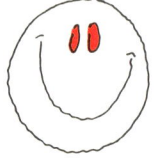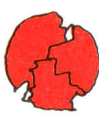

WARNING — take only as directed.

Rink-Dinks and Rinky-Dinkys

Directions: The answers to these riddles are two words that rhyme. The Rink-Dinks are one-syllable words; the Rinky-Dinkys, two-syllable words. Example of a Rink-Dink: What is an overweight rodent? Answer: A fat rat! If this is not the quiz for you, see page 39.

RINK-DINKS
1. What is Saturday for school children? _____
2. What is a smooth hen? _____
3. What is an irritated employer? _____
4. What is a joyful father? _____
5. What is a stupid friend? _____
6. What is an unusual seat? _____
7. What is a bashful insect? _____
8. What is a large hog? _____
9. What is an uncontrollable infant? _____
10. What is a fat fish? _____

RINKY-DINKYS
1. What is a beautiful cat? _____
2. What is a small skinny horse? _____
3. What is an attractive girl? _____
4. What is a comical rabbit? _____
5. What is a loafing flower? _____
6. What is a world of stone? _____

(See answers on pages 44-45.)

Fashion Plate's Designer Hospital Gown

No Well-Dressed Patient
Would Be Seen Without One

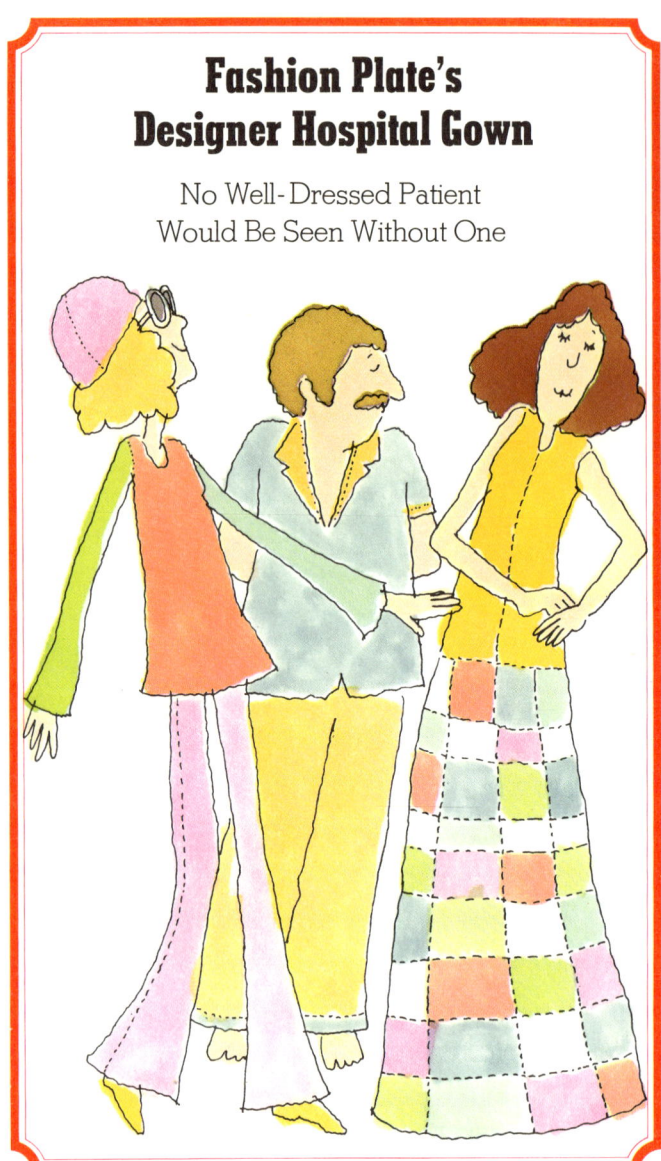

24

Directions:
1. Cut out the pieces of this pattern carefully and increase them 28½ times. The gown will fit a man weighing between 126 and 214 pounds and a woman weighing between 93 and 157 pounds.
2. Suggested materials: blue jean, pup tent, shower curtain, bottom sheet.
3. Sew this pattern as you would any other fine garment.
4. Due to the exclusiveness of this gown, we recommend that you only wear it for a short time.

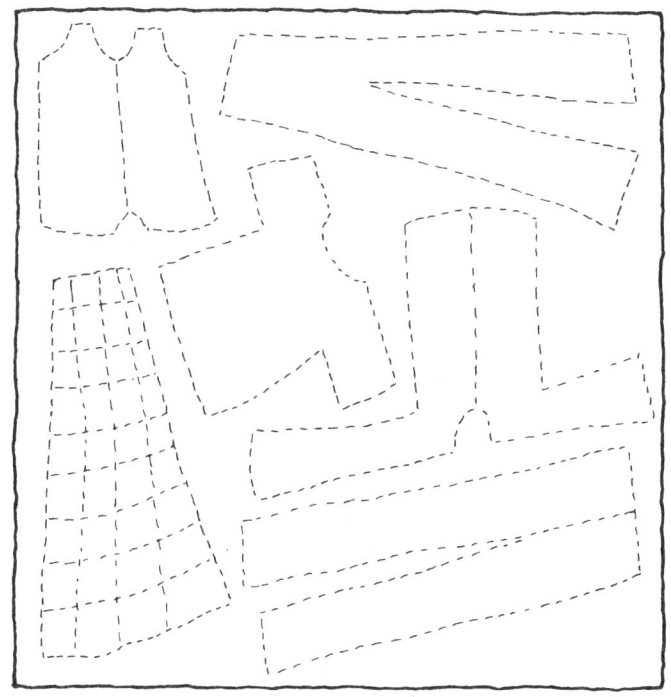

Dr. Don's
Daffy Jokes

Do you remember the story of the resourceful doctor who named his horse Consultation so his nurse could tell his patients, "Dr. Schmaltz can't see you this afternoon. He's out on Consultation"? Well, it's now proposed that the good doctor acquire a dog named Physician, so that, when subjecting the pooch to an obedience test, he can command, "Physician, heel thyself!"

A shipping tycoon, completing his annual physical checkup at a local hospital, was assured by the doctor in charge, "You're sound as a dollar, sir." The tycoon fainted.

The whole neighborhood shook from the explosion in the rear of the town's oldest pharmacy. The pharmacist himself staggered out, his glasses broken, streaks of black besmirching his white uniform. "Lady," he implored a customer who was wiping debris from the soda counter off herself, "would you please ask your doctor to copy off that prescription again — and this time I hope he'll PRINT it!"

The Word Tree
or If You Didn't Have a Problem, You've Got One Now

Directions:
Fill in blank spaces based on the clues given.
Example: (clue) Grand opening. (answer) Operation.
(See answers on page 45.)

1. Loves to needle you.
2. Under the weather.
3. Rough spot.
4. Something to duck.
5. Handles undercover work.
6. A cutup.
7. What doctors have.
8. Grand opening.
9. A sleeper.
10. Dracula's delight.

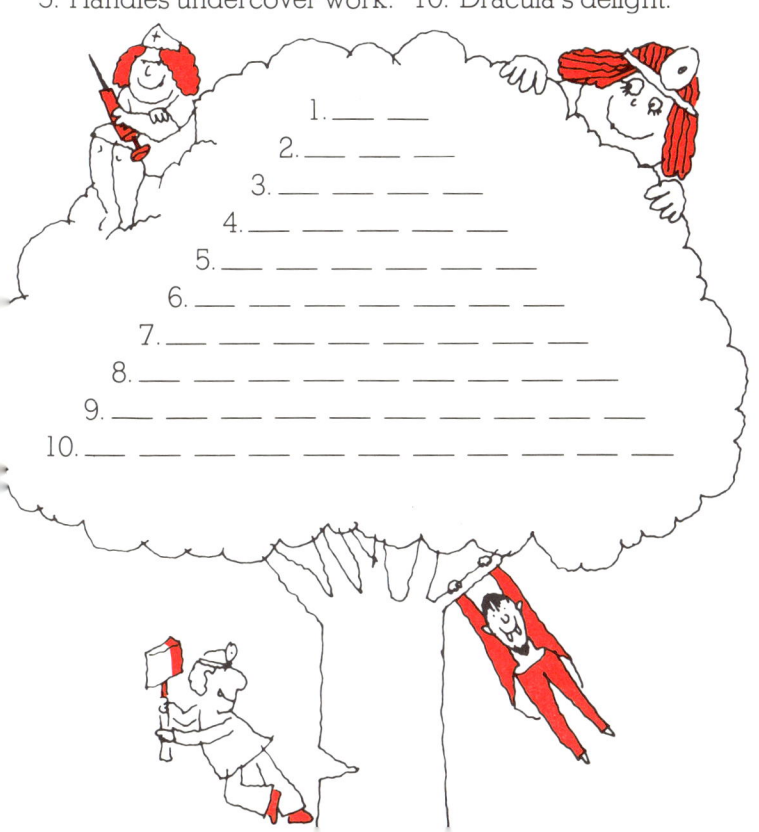

Doctor Horatio Neverfail's Handy Helpful Hints On How to Become The World's Most Remembered Patient

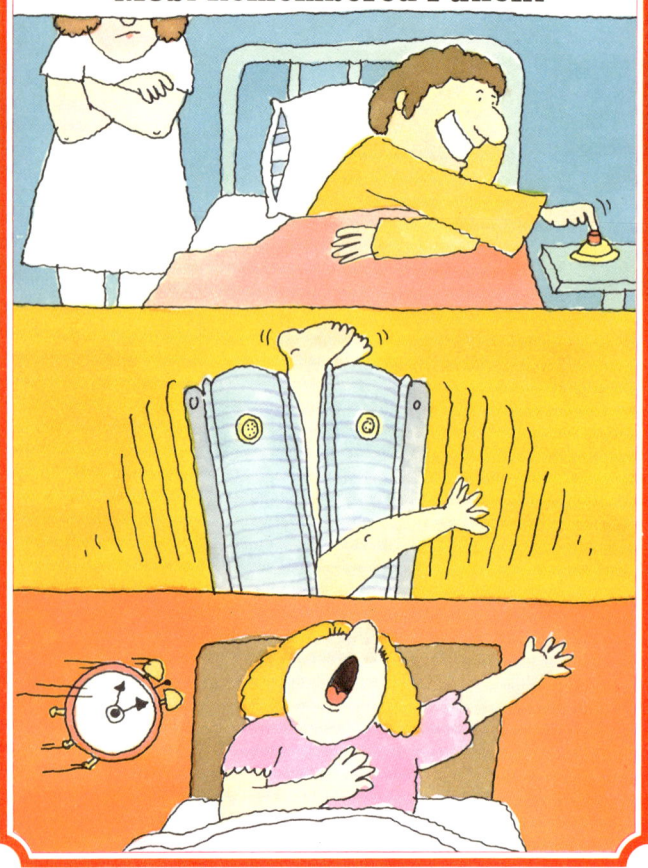

Let the Nurses Know You Like Them

Every fifteen minutes press the little button that lights up your room number at the nurses' station. You'll be surprised at how popular you'll become. All the nurses will be talking about how friendly you are, and you'll be sure to have lots of company.

Learn How Your Hospital Bed Works

A hospital bed is a fascinating piece of machinery. No use letting it just sit there unused. See how many different positions you can change it to in just ten minutes. The world professional bed-changing record is held by Craig Bendalot, famed sideshow double-jointed exhibitionist. The amateur record belongs to Malvina Sacrum, who entered the hospital with an ingrown toenail and worked her way up to a slipped disc by changing the angle of her bed 42½ times in ten minutes.

Learn to Yodel

Put your time to good use and make time pass quickly by learning a new skill. Learning to yodel is easy but requires much practice. The best time to practice is between 10 P.M. and midnight so you can hear all the subtle tonal inflections bounce off your walls. In no time at all you will hear sounds of appreciation from patients in all the other rooms on your floor.

Wonder Drugs

Wonder drugs are now in wide use. They are called wonder drugs because doctors wonder which one to prescribe and patients wonder how to pronounce them, why these drugs cost so much, and whether it is better to wake up every four hours during the night to take them or to get a good night's sleep.

Mention of wonder drugs calls to mind the pharmacist of today. He sells not only wonder drugs but ordinary drugs, as well as razor blades, alarm clocks, magazines, sunglasses, transistor radios, bathroom scales, greeting cards, candy, cigarettes, bedroom slippers, golf balls, and anything else you can think of. The pharmacist himself stays in the prescription room, performing mysterious rites such as scraping the label off a bottle and typing (with one finger, so as to be accurate) a label of his own.

The pharmacist is carefully trained to handle the complicated pharmaceuticals of today. In addition to learning how to pour from a wide-necked bottle into a narrow-necked bottle without spilling (the stuff is expensive), he must have the mathematical training to count as many as 100 pills and an even larger number of trading stamps. Another thing he is taught is to stay safely behind his bulletproof glass partition and let a clerk hand the filled prescription to the customer and tell how much it costs.

Richard Armour

Hey There — You With the Talent

Below are three facial outlines of a nurse and three of a doctor. For laughs, fill in the faces according to how our nurse and doctor look as they say:

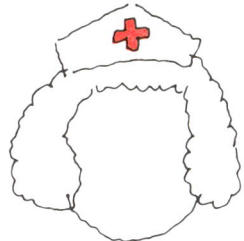
"Time for a bath."

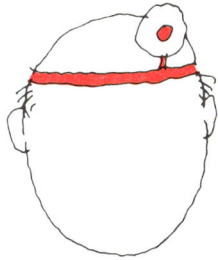
"Oh, you're not Mrs. Snatcher?"

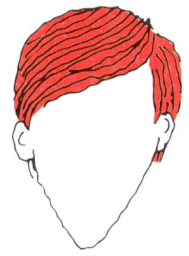
"The bedpan — again!"

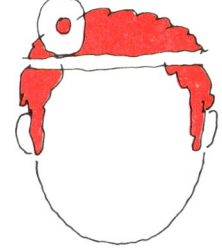
"This won't hurt at all."

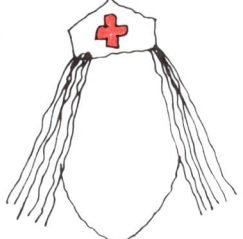
"But it's such a small hypo."

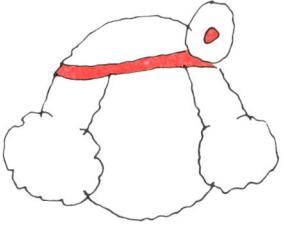
"Triplets!"

Lots of Quizzes

For your enjoyment, edification, enlightenment, endurance and they also give you something to do.

Vocabulary Quiz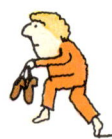

How many words of four or more letters can you find in the word below? Only one form of a word may be used. No proper names, please! Fifteen is good, twenty is excellent.

TIPTOED

History Quiz

Match each historical figure in Column A with the correct nickname in Column B.

A	B
1. Abe	a. The Terrible
2. Catherine	b. Queen of Scots
3. Andy Jackson	c. The Navigator
4. Cal	d. "Honest"
5. Eric	e. The Conqueror
6. Ivan	f. The Lionhearted
7. Mary	g. Old Hickory
8. Prince Henry	h. The Red
9. Richard	i. "Silent"
10. William	j. The Great

Literature Quiz

Using these clues, guess the last name of each famous literary figure.

1. Henry W. (Shortguy)
2. William (Rattleweapon)
3. John (Finished)
4. Robert (Scorches)
5. E. E. (Goings)
6. Robert (Chill)
7. Henry David (Exhaustive)
8. Elizabeth B. (Blueing)
9. Sara (Pestervalley)
10. Thomas (Weak)

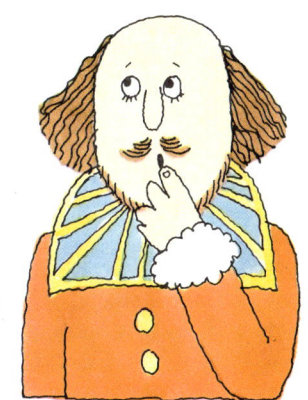

Art Lesson

Trace this without lifting your pencil from the page or retracing a line.

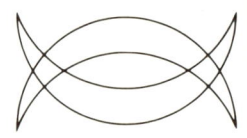

Join all the dots by making only four straight lines, and without lifting your pencil from the page.

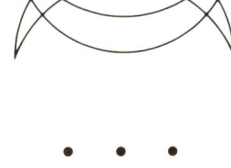

Draw this without lifting your pencil or retracing a line.

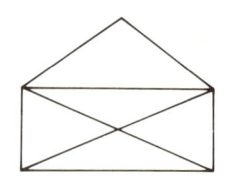

Geography Quiz

Using their abbreviations, which state is:

1. Oceangoing
2. Paternal
3. Egotistical
4. Astonished
5. Clean
6. Metallic
7. Professional
8. Sickly
9. Literary
10. Single

(See answers on pages 45-46.)

Some Proverbs to Cheer You

It is better to be well for two weeks than to be sick for a year.

When your temperature hits 100 — sell!

I'd rather be rich and healthy than poor and sick.

Sickness is a disease and should be treated as such.

Even the strongest person can become sick in a democracy.

An aspirin by any other name costs twice as much.

The best medicine nowadays costs no more than the cheapest nuclear submarine.

A stitch in time saves.

And last but not least — these famous words were uttered by a hypodermic-toting nurse in Cleveland:
It is better to give than to receive!

For the Business Mind

Here is a blank organization chart and a list of personnel who make up a typical hospital staff. Just for fun, use the chart to organize the staff for maximum efficiency. Be sure to pass this on to someone in charge. You won't get satin sheets or filet mignon for your efforts, but you might get a free operation (or at least an extra glass of orange juice).

Orderlies
Nurse's Aides
Nurses
Doctors
Cooks
Waker Uppers
Needle Sharpeners
Sterilizers
Interns
Outerns
Specimen Snatchers
Clothes Checkers
Bed Crankers
Food Tasters
Malnutricians
Electricians
Statisticians
Orange-Juice Pourers
Your Friendly Stork

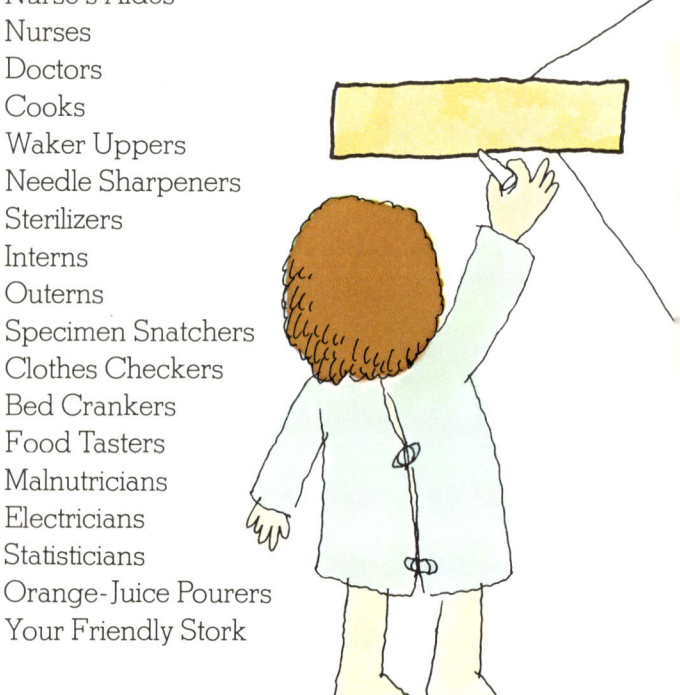

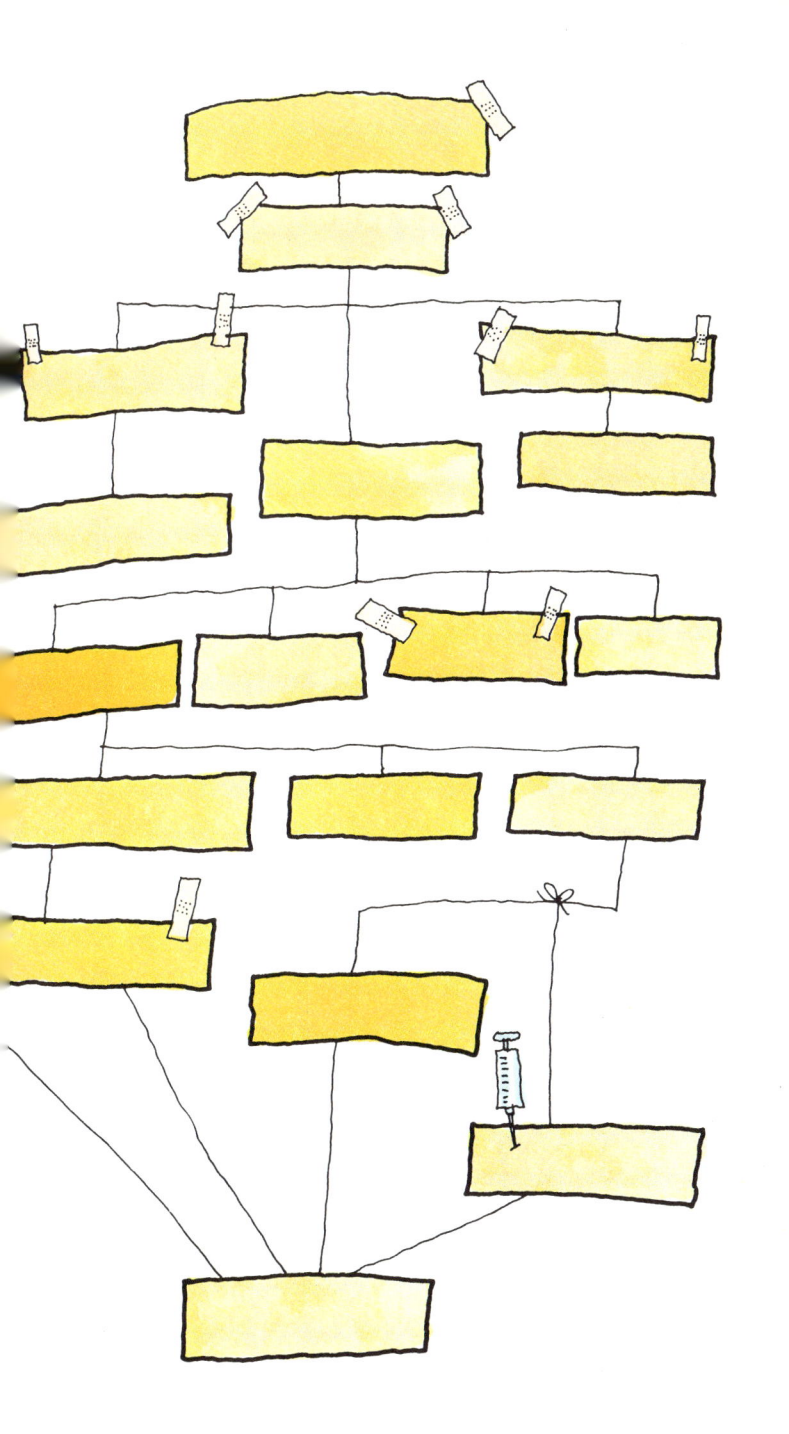

Joke Time

Hot chicken soup was the panacea for all illnesses, the elixir of life, the first and last resort. The humble chicken was our family's bluebird of happiness.

One of the classic stories... which has survived to this day — was about the mother who bought two live chickens. When she got home she discovered that one of the chickens was sick. She did then what any woman with a mother's heart would do — she killed the healthy chicken, made chicken soup, and fed it to the sick chicken. *Sam Levenson*

An eighty-year-old woman had just undergone a serious operation. Her doctor, following the rules of modern practice, told the nurse to get her out of bed and on her feet as soon as possible.

A few days after the operation, despite her obvious reluctance, the old lady was made to walk from her bed to a chair and back. Next day, still complaining, she was persuaded to walk around her room; still later she was marched up and down the hospital corridor. In a few weeks, she was discharged.

Not long afterward, her son called the doctor's office to tell him how delighted the whole family was at her recovery. "It was really remarkable," he exclaimed. "You know, Mother hadn't walked in five years!"

The _____ Quiz

Here is the quiz for people whose heads are filled with blanks. Complete the story by putting the correct words in the spaces provided. If this is not the quiz for you, see page 23.

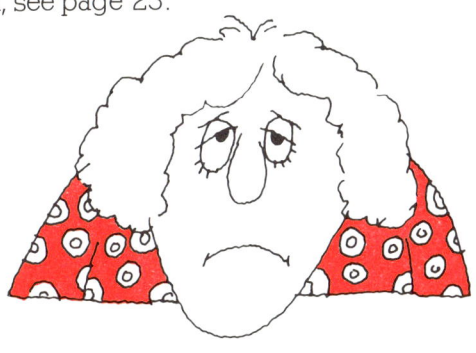

"From what you've told me," said the _____, "I'd say you need a complete _____. But let's have a look under your _____ first."

"Is that really necessary?" asked the _____.

"Yes," said the _____. "I want to see for myself what shape your _____ is in.

"Uh-huh! Just as I thought. From all indications, your _____ is run-down, your _____ is sluggish, and your _____ needs a complete cleaning out. But don't worry," he said, with a slap on the _____. "I'll have you running again smoothly in no time."

(See answers on page 46.)

For Those Who Are Mathematically Or Otherwise Inclined

Here are some riddles for the mathematical wizard as well as for those of us who must count on our fingers and toes whenever we balance our checkbook. Astound your friends and your sixth-grade arithmetic teacher by solving these problems.

1. Arrange the numbers from one to nine (inclusive) in a square like this so that the sum of the three numbers in each row, in each column, and along each diagonal will be fifteen.

2. Place four nines in such a way that the value expressed will be exactly one hundred.

3. Which is heavier, a pound of feathers or a pound of gold?

4. How long will it take a boy to cut a ten-foot pole into ten equal pieces if each cut takes one minute?

5. How many cubic feet of dirt are there in a hole which is a foot long, a foot wide, and a foot deep?

6. A boy has a box which contains just seven apples. He wishes to divide these apples among his seven friends so that each friend will get one apple and yet leave one apple in the box. How can this be done?

7. A snail starts at the bottom of a well twenty feet deep, crawls up four feet each day, and slips back three feet each night. How long will it take the snail to reach the top of the well?

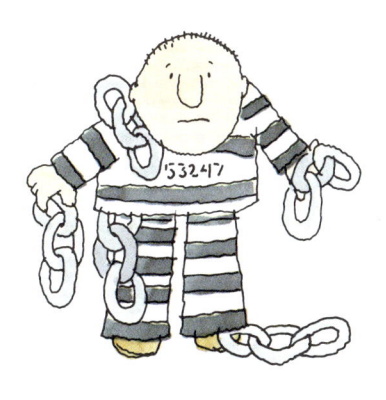

8. A man has five pieces of chain, each of which is made up of just three links. He wishes to have one chain made, using the five pieces. A blacksmith agrees to charge four cents for cutting a link and five cents for welding a link. What is the least amount for which the cutting and welding can be done?

(See answers on page 46.)

The Germ

A mighty creature is the germ,
Though smaller than the pachyderm.
His customary dwelling place
Is deep within the human race.
His childish pride he often pleases
By giving people strange diseases.
Do you, my poppet, feel infirm?
You probably contain a germ.

Ogden Nash

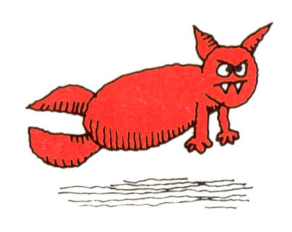

Answers
(So You Had to Look, Huh?)

Scramblers
1. With a SQUAWK
   laugh sweet taken quick
2. RECOVER
   wreck piker voice knock
3. Feeling GRAND
   gravy risky funny added
4. PERKY
   dirty broke penny chief
5. TICKLED
   black color adapt linen

Mystery Thrillers
1. Sharp knew that Pete McGee won the race because "he travels fastest who travels alone."
2. Sharp knew that "beggars can't be choosers."
3. Sharp said, "Your error was in naming this horse, for everyone knows that 'misery loves company.'"
4. Sharp knew that Sylvia Sweetsoul was the thief because she said she'd been with her best friend all day, and everyone knows that "diamonds are a girl's best friend."
5. Will and Phil could not have been lost, and Sharp knew it, for "where there's a *will* there's a way."

Personality Quiz
1. *Goat* — You're a crazy, mixed-up KID, but not a ba-a-a-d sort! *Rhinoceros* — You appear to be the thick-skinned type, but underneath it all you have a big heart! *Skunk* — You believe in the old adage "He travels fastest who travels alone," but there are still touches

of "SCENTIMENT" in your makeup! *Fox* — You're pretty FOXY aren't you, staying in bed all day? *Lion* — You're no doubt the aggressive type, which means you should soon ROAR OUT OF THERE!

2. *Southern Mansion* — Y'all enjoy easy livin'. You have a fondness for mint juleps, magnolias and homegrown tobacco. *Coed Dormitory* — You are definitely not chauvinistic in your preference of friends. *Lighthouse* — You are destined to be a GUIDING LIGHT in your community. *Neighborhood Bar* — Yesh shiree! You shirtainly couldn't have made a better choice! *Doghouse* — Okay, ROVER! Quit fooling around and get out of there.

3. *The Care and Cleaning of Fig Leaves* — You don't give a FIG for convention, but you take pride in your personal appearance. *How to Train a Sea Gull* — You crave companionship and you have a distinct liking for the name "JONATHAN." *The Life and Loves of Cleopatra* — Start digging! *Plantation Farming* — You're always looking for an opportunity to "raise cane"! *How to Build Your Own TV Set* — Hope you're UP AND OUT long before you'd have time to finish such a project!

4. *A pet yak* — You're quite a conversationalist, always YAKKING it up with friends. *A vacation* — Wouldn't we all? *A man* — You are a woman. *Money* — Wouldn't we all? *A woman* — You are a man.

Rink-Dinks 1. Play day   2. Slick chick   3. Cross boss
4. Glad dad   5. Dumb chum   6. Rare chair   7. Shy fly
8. Big pig   9. Wild child   10. Stout trout

Rinky-Dinkys 1. Pretty kitty 2. Bony pony
3. Classy lassie 4. Funny bunny 5. Lazy daisy
6. Granite planet

The Word Tree

```
         R   N
       I   L   L
     S   O   R   E
   Q   U   A   C   K
 B   E   D   P   A   N
S   U   R   G   E   O   N
P   A   T   I   E   N   T   S
O   P   E   R   A   T   I   O   N
A   N   E   S   T   H   E   T   I   C
T   R   A   N   S   F   U   S   I   O   N
```

Vocabulary Quiz

tepid	toed	tote	piet	potted	depot	doit
tide	topi	petit	pied	podite	diet	dote
tied	tope	pitted	poet	edit	ditto	dope

History Quiz
1. d 2. j 3. g 4. i 5. h 6. a 7. b 8. c 9. f 10. e

Literature Quiz
1. Longfellow 2. Shakespeare 3. Donne 4. Burns
5. Cummings 6. Frost 7. Thoreau 8. Browning
9. Teasdale 10. Hardy

Art Lesson

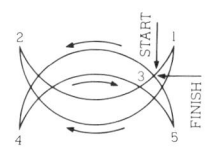

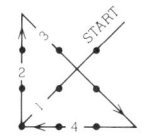

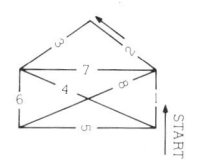